ACTIVE LIVING, HEALTHY LIFE

Managing Diabetes through Exercise

Richard Stone

TABLE OF CONTENTS

INTRODUCTION

Welcome to "Active Living, Healthy Life: Managing Diabetes through Exercise." In the modern world, where sedentary lifestyles and unhealthy eating habits prevail, the incidence of diabetes is on the rise. Diabetes, a chronic condition characterized by high blood sugar levels, can have significant impacts on an individual's health and quality of life. However, there is hope.

This book is a comprehensive guide that aims to explore the powerful connection between exercise and diabetes management. We will delve into the ways in which regular physical activity can play a pivotal role in regulating blood sugar levels, enhancing insulin sensitivity, and improving overall health for individuals living with diabetes.

Understanding the intricacies of diabetes is essential for effective management. We will begin by exploring the different types of diabetes, their causes, symptoms, and potential complications. Equipped with this knowledge, we will then embark on a journey to uncover the transformative potential of exercise.

The benefits of exercise for people with diabetes are multifaceted. By incorporating various types of physical activity into your daily routine, you can experience improvements in blood sugar control, cardiovascular health, weight management, and mental well-being. We will guide you through different forms of exercise, including aerobic exercises, strength training, and flexibility routines, helping you design a personalized exercise plan that suits your unique needs.

Moreover, we understand that exercise and diabetes management go hand in hand, and this book will shed light on the critical relationship between physical activity and blood sugar regulation. You will learn strategies to balance your blood sugar levels before, during, and after exercise, along with important considerations for adjusting diabetes medications and insulin dosages.

However, managing diabetes is not limited to exercise alone. We recognize the importance of a holistic approach to health and well-being. Throughout the book, we will explore the influence of lifestyle factors such as nutrition, hydration, stress management, and sleep on diabetes management.

We will also address common challenges faced by individuals with diabetes and provide practical tips for overcoming them. Additionally, inspiring case studies and success stories will motivate you on your journey to better health, showcasing how others have successfully managed their diabetes through exercise.

Whether you are newly diagnosed or have been living with diabetes for years, this book will equip you with the knowledge, tools, and inspiration to take control of your health. By empowering yourself with the information and strategies presented within these pages, you can embrace an active lifestyle and thrive in managing your diabetes.

Remember, exercise is not a burden but a powerful ally on your path to well-being. Together, let us embark on this transformative journey of exercise and diabetes management, reclaiming control of our health and living our best lives.

UNDERSTANDING DIABETES

In this chapter, we will lay the foundation for understanding diabetes. By gaining a comprehensive understanding of this condition, its types, causes, symptoms, and potential complications, you will be better equipped to appreciate the importance of exercise in managing diabetes effectively.

1. What is diabetes?

Diabetes is a chronic metabolic disorder characterized by elevated blood sugar levels. It occurs when the body either does not produce enough insulin (a hormone that regulates blood sugar) or cannot effectively use the insulin it produces. Insulin allows glucose (sugar) from the bloodstream to enter cells, where it is used for energy.

2. Types of diabetes (Type 1, Type 2, gestational diabetes):

Type 1 diabetes: This autoimmune condition typically develops in childhood or early adulthood. It occurs when the body's immune system mistakenly attacks and destroys the insulin-producing cells in the pancreas. As a result, individuals with Type 1 diabetes require lifelong insulin therapy.

Type 2 diabetes: The most common form of diabetes, Type 2, often develops later in life and is closely associated with lifestyle factors such as poor diet, sedentary behavior, and obesity. In Type 2 diabetes, the body becomes resistant to the effects of insulin or does not produce enough insulin.

Gestational diabetes: This type of diabetes occurs during pregnancy and affects the mother's ability to regulate blood sugar levels. Although it usually resolves after childbirth, women with gestational diabetes have an increased risk of developing Type 2 diabetes later in life.

3. Causes, symptoms, and complications of diabetes:

Causes: The causes of diabetes vary depending on the type. Type 1 diabetes is believed to have a genetic predisposition, while Type 2 diabetes is primarily influenced by lifestyle factors such as poor diet, physical inactivity, and obesity.

Gestational diabetes is thought to be related to hormonal changes during pregnancy.

Symptoms: Common symptoms of diabetes include increased thirst, frequent urination, unexplained weight loss, fatigue, blurred vision, and slow-healing wounds. However, some individuals may not experience noticeable symptoms, particularly in the early stages of Type 2 diabetes.

Complications: Poorly managed diabetes can lead to long-term complications such as cardiovascular disease, nerve damage, kidney disease, eye damage (retinopathy), foot problems, and an increased risk of infections.

4. Importance of diabetes management:

Diabetes management is crucial for preventing or minimizing the onset of complications associated with the condition. By effectively managing blood sugar levels, individuals with diabetes can reduce the risk of long-term health problems and enhance their overall well-being. Diabetes management encompasses various lifestyle modifications, including exercise, diet, medication, and regular monitoring of blood sugar levels.

Understanding the fundamentals of diabetes sets the stage for exploring the role of exercise in diabetes management. In the subsequent chapters, we will dive deeper into the transformative power of physical activity and learn how exercise can regulate blood sugar levels, improve insulin sensitivity, and empower individuals with diabetes to lead healthier lives.

EXERCISE AND DIABETES: THE POWERFUL DUO

In this chapter, we will explore the profound connection between exercise and diabetes management. Regular physical activity has been shown to have remarkable benefits for individuals living with diabetes, from controlling blood sugar levels to improving overall health and well-being. By understanding the role of exercise in diabetes management, you will be inspired to incorporate physical activity into your daily routine and reap its countless rewards.

1. The role of exercise in diabetes management:

Exercise plays a crucial role in effectively managing diabetes. It helps regulate blood sugar levels, enhances insulin sensitivity, and reduces insulin resistance. Engaging in regular physical activity is a powerful tool for individuals with diabetes to maintain optimal health and prevent complications associated with the condition.

2. How exercise affects blood sugar levels:

During exercise, muscles require energy, which is predominantly supplied by glucose from the bloodstream. As a result, blood sugar levels decrease as glucose is utilized for energy. Regular exercise also improves the body's overall ability to control blood sugar levels, leading to more stable and balanced glucose readings over time.

3. Benefits of exercise for individuals with diabetes:

Exercise offers numerous benefits for individuals living with diabetes, including:

- ➢ Improved blood sugar control: Regular physical activity helps to lower and stabilize blood sugar levels, reducing the need for medication or insulin.

- ➢ Weight management: Exercise aids in weight loss or weight maintenance, which is particularly important for individuals with Type 2 diabetes as obesity is a risk factor for the condition.

- ➢ Cardiovascular health: Physical activity strengthens the heart, improves circulation, and lowers the risk of cardiovascular diseases, which are more prevalent in individuals with diabetes.

➢ Insulin sensitivity: Exercise enhances the body's response to insulin, making it more effective in transporting glucose into cells, thus improving insulin sensitivity.

➢ Stress reduction: Exercise has been shown to reduce stress levels and improve mental well-being, which is beneficial for managing diabetes as stress can impact blood sugar control.

➢ Enhanced overall fitness: Regular exercise improves stamina, muscle strength, flexibility, and overall fitness levels, contributing to a healthier and more active lifestyle.

4. Exercise guidelines for people with diabetes:

To maximize the benefits of exercise and ensure safety, individuals with diabetes should follow specific guidelines:

➢ Consult with a healthcare professional: Before starting an exercise program, it is essential to consult with a healthcare provider to assess individual fitness levels, consider any complications, and tailor the exercise plan accordingly.

➢ Choose appropriate exercises: Incorporate a variety of aerobic, strength training, flexibility, and balance exercises into your routine.

➢ Start gradually and progress slowly: Begin with low-impact exercises and gradually increase intensity, duration, and frequency over time.

➢ Monitor blood sugar levels: Regularly check blood sugar levels before, during, and after exercise to understand the impact of physical activity on blood sugar control.

➢ Stay hydrated: Maintain proper hydration before, during, and after exercise to support optimal performance and prevent dehydration.

➢ Consider safety precautions: Be aware of potential risks such as hypoglycemia (low blood sugar) and take necessary precautions to manage them effectively.

By recognizing the profound benefits of exercise for individuals with diabetes and adhering to appropriate guidelines, you can harness the power of physical activity to effectively manage your condition and improve your overall health. In the following chapters, we will delve deeper into different types of exercise, tailor an exercise plan for diabetes management, and explore the intricate relationship between exercise and blood sugar regulation.

TYPES OF EXERCISE FOR DIABETES MANAGEMENT

In this chapter, we will explore various types of exercises that are beneficial for diabetes management. Engaging in a well-rounded exercise routine that includes aerobic exercises, strength training exercises, flexibility exercises, and balance exercises can provide comprehensive health benefits and contribute to improved blood sugar control. By understanding and incorporating these different types of exercises, you can optimize your diabetes management and enhance your overall well-being.

1. Aerobic exercises:

Aerobic exercises, also known as cardiovascular exercises, are activities that increase your heart rate and breathing rate. These exercises are essential for managing diabetes as they help improve insulin sensitivity, burn calories, and control blood sugar levels. Examples of aerobic exercises include:

➢ Walking: Walking is a low-impact exercise that can be easily incorporated into your daily routine. It improves cardiovascular fitness and is accessible to people of various fitness levels.

➢ Cycling: Whether outdoors or using a stationary bike, cycling is a great aerobic exercise that strengthens the legs, improves cardiovascular health, and burns calories.

➢ Swimming: Swimming is a low-impact exercise that is gentle on the joints. It provides a full-body workout, improves cardiovascular fitness, and helps build strength and endurance.

➢ Dancing: Dancing is a fun and engaging way to get your heart pumping. It can be done in various forms such as Zumba, salsa, or ballroom dancing, offering both physical and mental benefits.

2. Strength training exercises:

Strength training exercises involve working against resistance to build muscle strength and endurance. These exercises are crucial for diabetes management as they help increase muscle mass, improve insulin sensitivity, and enhance overall metabolism. Examples of strength training exercises include:

> Weightlifting: Using dumbbells, barbells, or resistance machines, weightlifting exercises target specific muscle groups and help build strength and muscle mass.

> Bodyweight exercises: Exercises such as push-ups, squats, lunges, and planks use your body weight as resistance and can be performed anywhere without the need for equipment.

> Resistance band exercises: Resistance bands are portable and versatile tools that provide resistance for strength training exercises. They are suitable for all fitness levels and can target different muscle groups.

3. Flexibility and balance exercises:

Flexibility and balance exercises are essential for maintaining joint mobility, preventing injuries, and improving overall functional ability. These exercises are particularly important for individuals with diabetes, as they can help improve posture, reduce muscle imbalances, and enhance overall movement quality. Examples of flexibility and balance exercises include:

> Yoga: Yoga combines stretching, strength, and balance exercises, promoting flexibility, relaxation, and mind-body connection.

> Pilates: Pilates focuses on core strength, flexibility, and body awareness. It incorporates controlled movements and breathing techniques to improve posture and overall body alignment.

> Tai Chi: Tai Chi is a gentle and slow-moving exercise that improves balance, flexibility, and mental relaxation. It involves a series of flowing movements and is suitable for individuals of all ages and fitness levels.

By incorporating a combination of aerobic exercises, strength training exercises, flexibility exercises, and balance exercises into your routine, you can experience comprehensive health benefits and optimize your diabetes management. In the upcoming chapters, we will discuss how to tailor an exercise plan that suits your individual needs, setting realistic goals, and tracking your progress along the way.

TAILORING AN EXERCISE PLAN FOR DIABETES

In this chapter, we will guide you through the process of tailoring an exercise plan specifically designed for managing diabetes. Recognizing that every individual has unique needs, abilities, and preferences, we will explore how to assess your fitness level, set realistic goals, and create a personalized exercise routine that is sustainable and effective. By following these guidelines, you will be able to establish an exercise plan that empowers you to regulate your blood sugar levels and improve your overall health and well-being.

1. Assessing individual fitness level and goals:

Before embarking on any exercise program, it is essential to assess your current fitness level and identify your goals. This assessment will help you gauge your starting point and establish a baseline for progress. Consider the following factors:

- Medical history: Take into account any existing health conditions, injuries, or physical limitations that may affect your exercise choices.

- Physical abilities: Assess your current fitness level, including cardiovascular endurance, strength, flexibility, and balance.

- Blood sugar control: Evaluate how well your blood sugar levels are managed and any patterns or challenges you may have noticed during physical activity.

- Personal preferences: Consider your interests, lifestyle, and availability of resources to select activities that you enjoy and can realistically incorporate into your routine.

- Short-term and long-term goals: Set specific, measurable, attainable, relevant, and time-bound (SMART) goals that align with your overall diabetes management objectives.

2. Designing an exercise plan based on personal needs:

Once you have assessed your fitness level and identified your goals, it's time to design an exercise plan tailored to your individual needs. Consider the following aspects:

- ➤ Exercise frequency: Determine how many days per week you can commit to exercise. Aim for a minimum of 150 minutes of moderate-intensity aerobic activity or 75 minutes of vigorous-intensity aerobic activity spread across the week, along with strength training exercises at least twice a week.

- ➤ Exercise duration: Gradually increase the duration of your exercise sessions. Start with shorter durations and gradually work your way up to longer sessions as your fitness level improves.

- ➤ Exercise intensity: Choose exercises that allow you to work at a moderate intensity, where you feel slightly out of breath but can still carry on a conversation. However, consult with your healthcare provider to establish appropriate intensity levels based on your specific needs.

➤ Exercise type: Select a combination of aerobic exercises, strength training exercises, flexibility exercises, and balance exercises that align with your interests and goals.

➤ Progression and variety: Regularly reassess your fitness level and modify your exercise routine to ensure continued progress and prevent boredom. Incorporate new activities or increase the intensity or duration of your existing exercises to challenge your body.

3. Setting realistic goals and tracking progress:

Setting realistic goals is crucial for maintaining motivation and tracking progress. Consider the following strategies:

➤ SMART goals: Set specific, measurable, attainable, relevant, and time-bound goals that align with your overall diabetes management objectives.

➢ Track your progress: Keep a record of your exercise sessions, including duration, intensity, and any observations related to blood sugar levels. Use a fitness tracker or journal to monitor your progress and celebrate your achievements.

➢ Celebrate milestones: Acknowledge and reward yourself for reaching milestones along the way. This can help maintain motivation and provide a sense of accomplishment.

4. Creating an exercise routine that is sustainable:

To ensure long-term success, it's important to create an exercise routine that is sustainable and enjoyable. Consider the following tips:

➢ Mix it up: Incorporate a variety of exercises to keep your routine interesting and engaging. This can include outdoor activities, group classes, or trying new workout formats.

➢ Find a workout buddy or join a community: Exercising with a partner or joining a fitness community can provide support, motivation, and accountability.

- ➢ Listen to your body: Pay attention to how your body responds to exercise. If you experience pain, discomfort, or unusual symptoms, consult with your healthcare provider and modify your exercise routine as necessary.
- ➢ Adapt to changes: Be flexible and adapt your exercise routine to accommodate changes in your schedule, physical abilities, or preferences.

By tailoring an exercise plan that suits your individual needs, setting realistic goals, and tracking your progress, you will be able to effectively manage your diabetes through exercise. In the subsequent chapters, we will delve deeper into the intricacies of blood sugar regulation during exercise, provide tips for safe and effective workouts, and explore ways to overcome common challenges faced by individuals with diabetes.

BLOOD SUGAR REGULATION DURING EXERCISE

In this chapter, we will explore the intricate relationship between exercise and blood sugar regulation in individuals with diabetes. Understanding how different types and intensities of exercise affect blood sugar levels is crucial for safe and effective diabetes management. By delving into the mechanisms behind blood sugar regulation during exercise and learning practical strategies to prevent hypoglycemia (low blood sugar) and hyperglycemia (high blood sugar), you will be better equipped to navigate the challenges and optimize the benefits of exercise for your diabetes management.

1. How exercise affects blood sugar levels:

During exercise, muscles require energy to perform the physical activity. As a result, the body releases stored glucose from the liver and increases the uptake of glucose from the bloodstream into the muscles. This leads to a decrease in blood sugar levels during and after exercise. However, the impact of exercise on blood sugar levels can vary depending on several factors, including the type, intensity, and duration of exercise, as well as individual factors such as medication use and diet.

2. Preventing hypoglycemia during exercise:

Hypoglycemia, characterized by low blood sugar levels, is a potential risk during exercise for individuals with diabetes. To prevent hypoglycemia, consider the following strategies:

> Blood sugar monitoring: Regularly check your blood sugar levels before, during, and after exercise to understand how your body responds to different activities. This will help you make informed decisions about managing your blood sugar during exercise.

> Adjusting medication and carbohydrate intake: Depending on your medication regimen and individual needs, you may need to adjust your medication doses and carbohydrate intake before and during exercise to maintain stable blood sugar

levels. Consult with your healthcare provider for personalized guidance.

➢ Snacking before and during exercise: Consuming a small snack that combines carbohydrates and protein before exercise can help prevent hypoglycemia. Additionally, for longer or more intense workouts, consider consuming carbohydrates during exercise to sustain blood sugar levels.

➢ Carrying glucose or fast-acting carbohydrates: Always have a source of glucose or fast-acting carbohydrates readily available during exercise in case of hypoglycemia. This can be in the form of glucose tablets, fruit juice, or other quick-acting carbohydrates.

3. Managing hyperglycemia during exercise:

Hyperglycemia, characterized by high blood sugar levels, can also occur during exercise, particularly if blood sugar levels are already elevated before starting physical activity.

To manage hyperglycemia during exercise, consider the following strategies:

- ➢ Regular blood sugar monitoring: Monitor your blood sugar levels before, during, and after exercise to identify any patterns of hyperglycemia. This information will help you adjust your medication, carbohydrate intake, and exercise routine as needed.

- ➢ Ensuring proper hydration: Stay well-hydrated before, during, and after exercise. Dehydration can contribute to higher blood sugar levels. Drink plenty of water and avoid sugary drinks that can further elevate blood sugar levels.

- ➢ Adjusting medication and insulin doses: Consult with your healthcare provider about adjusting your medication or insulin doses to better manage blood sugar levels during exercise. Timing and dosing adjustments may be necessary for certain individuals.

- ➢ Choosing appropriate exercise intensity: Engage in moderate-intensity exercises that allow you to maintain a comfortable level of exertion without overexerting yourself. High-intensity exercise can sometimes lead to temporary spikes in blood sugar levels.

4. Safety precautions during exercise:

In addition to managing blood sugar levels, it's important to take general safety precautions during exercise. Consider the following:

- ➤ Wear medical identification: Always wear a medical identification bracelet or carry a card that indicates you have diabetes. This will provide important information to healthcare professionals in case of an emergency.
- ➤ Stay hydrated: Drink plenty of water before, during, and after exercise to prevent dehydration, which can affect blood sugar control and overall performance.
- ➤ Protect your feet: Individuals with diabetes may be more prone to foot-related complications. Ensure

you wear proper footwear and regularly inspect your feet for any signs of injury or infection.

➢ Be mindful of environmental conditions: Extreme temperatures, both hot and cold, can affect blood sugar control. Take necessary precautions to protect yourself from extreme weather conditions.

By understanding the intricacies of blood sugar regulation during exercise and implementing practical strategies to prevent hypoglycemia and manage hyperglycemia, you can safely and effectively incorporate exercise into your diabetes management routine. In the upcoming chapters, we will provide guidance on creating a safe workout environment, offer exercise tips for specific diabetes types, and explore strategies for overcoming common exercise barriers faced by individuals with diabetes.

CREATING A SAFE EXERCISE ENVIRONMENT FOR DIABETES

In this chapter, we will delve into the importance of creating a safe exercise environment when managing diabetes. Engaging in physical activity in a supportive and safe setting is essential for optimizing the benefits of exercise while minimizing potential risks. We will explore key considerations for creating a safe exercise environment, including managing blood sugar levels, ensuring proper equipment and attire, and understanding the importance of warming up and cooling down. By implementing these strategies, you can exercise with confidence, knowing that you are taking the necessary precautions to prioritize your well-being.

1. Managing blood sugar levels before exercise:

Before starting any exercise session, it is crucial to ensure that your blood sugar levels are within a safe range. Consider the following guidelines:

➤ Check your blood sugar levels: Monitor your blood sugar levels before exercising. If your levels are too high or too low, take appropriate steps to bring them into a safe range before engaging in physical activity.

➤ Adjust your medication and carbohydrate intake: Depending on your individual needs and medication regimen, you may need to adjust your medication or carbohydrate intake to maintain stable blood sugar levels during exercise. Consult with your healthcare provider for personalized guidance.

2. Proper equipment and attire:

Using appropriate equipment and wearing suitable attire can contribute to a safe and comfortable exercise experience. Consider the following recommendations:

➤ Footwear: Wear well-fitting, supportive shoes that provide stability and cushioning. Proper footwear is particularly important for individuals with diabetes, as it can help prevent foot injuries and complications.

➢ Comfortable clothing: Choose breathable, moisture-wicking fabrics that allow for freedom of movement. Dress in layers to accommodate changes in temperature during exercise.

➢ Safety accessories: If engaging in outdoor activities, wear reflective gear or bright colors to enhance visibility, especially during low-light conditions. Additionally, consider wearing a helmet for activities such as cycling or skating to protect against head injuries.

3. Warming up and cooling down:

Performing warm-up and cool-down exercises before and after your workout sessions is essential for injury prevention and overall safety. Consider the following practices:

➢ Warm-up: Begin your exercise session with a 5 to 10-minute warm-up that includes dynamic stretching and low-intensity movements. This helps increase blood flow, loosen up muscles, and prepare your body for the upcoming workout.

➤ Cool-down: Conclude your exercise session with a 5 to 10-minute cool-down, which includes gentle stretching and low-intensity movements. This helps gradually lower your heart rate, prevent dizziness or fainting, and promote recovery.

4. Safety considerations for different exercise settings:

The safety considerations may vary depending on the exercise setting. Consider the following guidelines:

➤ Gym or fitness center: Familiarize yourself with the equipment and ask for guidance from fitness professionals if needed. Clean and sanitize the equipment before use, and ensure proper form and technique to avoid injuries.

➤ Outdoor activities: If exercising outdoors, be mindful of your surroundings, including traffic, uneven surfaces, and potential hazards. Stay hydrated, protect yourself from extreme weather conditions, and consider carrying a form of identification that indicates you have diabetes.

> ➤ Group classes or sports: Choose classes or sports activities that are appropriate for your fitness level and skill set. Inform instructors or coaches about your diabetes and any specific considerations they should be aware of. Keep fast-acting carbohydrates readily available in case of hypoglycemia.

By creating a safe exercise environment that prioritizes blood sugar management, proper equipment and attire, warm-up and cool-down routines, and considering safety considerations for different exercise settings, you can reduce the risk of injuries and complications while maximizing the benefits of physical activity. In the following chapters, we will provide exercise recommendations for specific diabetes types, address common exercise barriers, and offer strategies to maintain long-term adherence to an active lifestyle.

EXERCISE RECOMMENDATIONS FOR DIFFERENT DIABETES TYPES

In this chapter, we will explore exercise recommendations tailored to different types of diabetes, including type 1 diabetes, type 2 diabetes, and gestational diabetes. Each type of diabetes presents unique considerations and challenges when it comes to exercise. By understanding these nuances and implementing appropriate strategies, you can effectively manage your diabetes while reaping the numerous benefits of physical activity. We will delve into specific exercise recommendations, precautions, and considerations for each diabetes type to help you make informed decisions about your exercise routine.

1. Exercise for Type 1 Diabetes:

Type 1 diabetes is characterized by the body's inability to produce insulin. When engaging in exercise, individuals with type 1 diabetes need to consider the following:

➢ Blood sugar monitoring: Regularly monitor your blood sugar levels before, during, and after exercise to understand how your body responds to different activities. This will help you make informed decisions about managing your blood sugar during exercise.

➤ Adjusting insulin doses: Depending on the intensity and duration of exercise, you may need to adjust your insulin doses to prevent hypoglycemia. Consult with your healthcare provider for personalized guidance on insulin adjustments.

➤ Carbohydrate intake: Consume carbohydrates before, during, or after exercise as needed to maintain stable blood sugar levels. It may be helpful to experiment with different carbohydrate sources and timing to find what works best for you.

➤ Hypoglycemia prevention: Be prepared to treat and prevent hypoglycemia by carrying fast-acting carbohydrates or glucose tablets during exercise.

2. Exercise for Type 2 Diabetes:

Type 2 diabetes is characterized by insulin resistance, where the body does not effectively use insulin. When incorporating exercise into your routine as someone with type 2 diabetes, consider the following recommendations:

- ➤ Consult with your healthcare provider: Discuss your exercise plans with your healthcare provider to ensure they are appropriate for your individual needs and medical condition.

- ➤ Blood sugar monitoring: Regularly monitor your blood sugar levels to assess how exercise affects your levels and adjust your medication or carbohydrate intake accordingly.

- ➤ Focus on aerobic and resistance exercises: Engage in a combination of aerobic exercises, such as walking, swimming, or cycling, and resistance exercises, such as weightlifting or bodyweight exercises. This can help improve insulin sensitivity, manage weight, and enhance overall fitness.

- ➤ Gradual progression: Start with low-impact activities and gradually increase the intensity and duration of your workouts. This allows your body to adapt and reduces the risk of injury.

➢ Aim for consistency: Strive for regular exercise, aiming for at least 150 minutes of moderate-intensity aerobic activity per week, along with strength training exercises at least twice a week.

5. Exercise for Gestational Diabetes:

Gestational diabetes occurs during pregnancy and can increase the risk of complications for both the mother and the baby. When incorporating exercise into your routine as someone with gestational diabetes, consider the following recommendations:

➢ Consult with your healthcare provider: Before starting any exercise program, consult with your healthcare provider to ensure it is safe and suitable for your specific situation.

➢ Blood sugar monitoring: Regularly monitor your blood sugar levels before, during, and after exercise to understand how your body responds. This will help you make adjustments to maintain stable blood sugar levels.

> Low-impact activities: Opt for low-impact exercises such as walking, swimming, or prenatal yoga, which are generally safe during pregnancy. Avoid activities that carry a high risk of falls or abdominal trauma.

> Stay hydrated: Drink plenty of water before, during, and after exercise to stay hydrated, as dehydration can affect blood sugar control and overall health.

> Listen to your body: Pay attention to any signs of discomfort or fatigue during exercise and adjust your activity level or intensity accordingly.

By considering the specific recommendations for each type of diabetes and working closely with your healthcare provider, you can safely and effectively incorporate exercise into your diabetes management routine. In the upcoming chapters, we will address common exercise barriers, provide strategies for maintaining long-term adherence, and explore additional considerations for exercise and diabetes management.

OVERCOMING COMMON EXERCISE BARRIERS FOR DIABETES MANAGEMENT

While exercise offers numerous benefits for diabetes management, it is not without its challenges. In this chapter, we will discuss common exercise barriers faced by individuals with diabetes and provide strategies to overcome them. By addressing these barriers head-on, you can develop strategies to maintain a consistent exercise routine, improve your overall health, and effectively manage your diabetes. Whether it's lack of motivation, time constraints, fear of hypoglycemia, or other obstacles, we will explore practical solutions to help you overcome these challenges and stay on track with your exercise goals.

1. Lack of Motivation:

Finding the motivation to exercise regularly can be challenging for anyone. Consider the following strategies to overcome a lack of motivation:

> Set realistic goals: Establish achievable short-term and long-term goals that are specific, measurable,

attainable, relevant, and time-bound (SMART goals). Break down larger goals into smaller milestones to track progress and stay motivated.

➤ Find activities you enjoy: Engage in activities that you find enjoyable and fulfilling. Experiment with different types of exercises and find what resonates with you. This can make exercise feel less like a chore and more like an enjoyable part of your daily routine.

➤ Buddy up: Find a workout partner or join a fitness community to stay motivated and accountable. Exercising with others can make the experience more enjoyable and provide an extra level of support.

2. Time Constraints:

Busy schedules and competing priorities can make it difficult to find time for exercise. Consider the following strategies to overcome time constraints:

➤ Prioritize physical activity: Make exercise a non-negotiable part of your daily routine by scheduling it into your calendar. Treat it as an essential self-care activity that deserves dedicated time.

➢ Break it up: If finding a continuous block of time for exercise is challenging, break it up into smaller bouts throughout the day. Even short bursts of activity, such as a 10-minute walk after each meal, can add up to significant health benefits.

➢ Multitask: Look for opportunities to incorporate physical activity into your daily activities. For example, take the stairs instead of the elevator, walk or bike to nearby destinations instead of driving, or use exercise equipment while watching TV or reading.

3. Fear of Hypoglycemia:

Fear of hypoglycemia (low blood sugar) can be a significant concern for individuals with diabetes when engaging in physical activity. Consider the following strategies to overcome this fear:

> Blood sugar monitoring: Regularly monitor your blood sugar levels before, during, and after exercise to understand how your body responds. This information will help you make informed decisions about managing your blood sugar during exercise.

> Pre-exercise snack: Consume a small snack containing carbohydrates and protein before exercising to prevent hypoglycemia. Adjust the timing and content of your snack based on your individual needs and blood sugar responses.

> Carry fast-acting carbohydrates: Keep a source of glucose or fast-acting carbohydrates readily available during exercise in case of hypoglycemia. This can provide reassurance and prompt treatment if needed.

4. Exercise-related Injuries:

Concerns about potential injuries can deter some individuals from engaging in exercise. Consider the following strategies to prevent injuries and alleviate concerns:

- ➢ Consult with a healthcare professional: Before starting any exercise program, consult with a healthcare professional or an exercise specialist to ensure you are engaging in safe and appropriate activities for your fitness level and medical condition.

- ➢ Start slow and progress gradually: Begin with low-impact activities and gradually increase the intensity and duration of your workouts. This allows your body to adapt and reduces the risk of overuse injuries.

- ➢ Focus on proper form and technique: Learn and practice proper form and technique for each exercise to minimize the risk of injuries. Consider working with a certified fitness professional for guidance.

By addressing common exercise barriers, such as lack of motivation, time constraints, fear of hypoglycemia, and exercise-related injuries, you can overcome these challenges and establish a sustainable exercise routine for managing your diabetes. In the following chapters, we will delve into additional considerations, including nutrition for exercise, mental well-being, and long-term adherence strategies for maintaining an active and healthy lifestyle with diabetes.

NUTRITION FOR EXERCISE AND DIABETES MANAGEMENT

Proper nutrition plays a vital role in supporting exercise performance, optimizing blood sugar control, and overall diabetes management. In this chapter, we will explore the relationship between nutrition, exercise, and diabetes, providing practical guidelines for fueling your workouts, managing blood sugar levels, and promoting overall health. From pre-exercise meals to post-workout recovery, we will delve into the key components of a balanced and diabetes-friendly nutrition plan to support your exercise routine and enhance your well-being.

1. Pre-Exercise Nutrition:

Fueling your body with the right nutrients before exercise is crucial for maintaining energy levels and preventing blood sugar imbalances. Consider the following guidelines:

- ➤ Timing: Consume a pre-exercise meal or snack 1-3 hours before your workout to provide your body with the necessary fuel without causing discomfort during exercise.

- ➢ Carbohydrates: Include a moderate amount of carbohydrates in your pre-exercise meal or snack. Opt for complex carbohydrates such as whole grains, fruits, and vegetables, as they provide sustained energy release.
- ➢ Protein: Include a source of lean protein in your pre-exercise meal or snack to support muscle repair and recovery. Good options include lean meats, fish, poultry, legumes, or dairy products.
- ➢ Hydration: Ensure adequate hydration before exercise by drinking water or consuming hydrating beverages. Avoid excessive caffeine or sugary drinks that can affect blood sugar control.

2. During-Exercise Nutrition:

For longer-duration or intense workouts, it may be necessary to consume additional nutrients during exercise to sustain energy levels and prevent hypoglycemia. Consider the following strategies:

> Carbohydrate intake: Depending on the duration and intensity of your exercise, consume carbohydrates during your workout to maintain blood sugar levels. This can be in the form of sports drinks, gels, or easily digestible snacks like fruit or granola bars.

> Blood sugar monitoring: Regularly check your blood sugar levels during longer workouts to ensure they stay within a safe range. Adjust your carbohydrate intake accordingly.

> Hydration: Stay hydrated during exercise by sipping on water or electrolyte-rich fluids. Consider the use of sugar-free electrolyte drinks for replenishing electrolytes lost through sweat.

3. Post-Exercise Recovery Nutrition:

Proper post-workout nutrition is essential for muscle recovery, glycogen replenishment, and overall recovery. Consider the following recommendations:

➢ Timing: Consume a post-workout meal or snack within 30-60 minutes after exercise to optimize recovery.

➢ Protein: Include a source of high-quality protein in your post-workout meal or snack to support muscle repair and growth. Options include lean meats, fish, poultry, eggs, dairy products, or plant-based protein sources.

➢ Carbohydrates: Include a moderate amount of carbohydrates in your post-workout meal or snack to replenish glycogen stores and support recovery. Opt for a mix of complex carbohydrates and a small amount of simple carbohydrates to promote faster glycogen replenishment.

➢ Hydration: Rehydrate by drinking water or electrolyte-rich fluids after exercise to replace fluids lost through sweating.

4. Blood Sugar Management During Exercise:

Proper blood sugar management is crucial when exercising with diabetes. Consider the following strategies:

- Blood sugar monitoring: Regularly monitor your blood sugar levels before, during, and after exercise to understand how your body responds. This information will help you make necessary adjustments to your nutrition and medication if needed.

- Adjusting insulin doses: Depending on your blood sugar levels and the intensity of your exercise, you may need to adjust your insulin doses. Work with your healthcare provider to develop a personalized plan for insulin adjustments during exercise.

- Carbohydrate counting: Learn to count carbohydrates in your meals and snacks to determine the amount of insulin or oral diabetes medications needed to maintain blood sugar control during exercise.

➢ Individualized approach: Diabetes management is highly individualized. Experiment with different approaches to nutrition and blood sugar management during exercise to find what works best for you. Consult with your healthcare provider or a registered dietitian for personalized guidance.

By implementing sound nutrition strategies before, during, and after exercise, you can optimize your performance, maintain stable blood sugar levels, and support overall diabetes management. In the next chapter, we will explore the importance of mental well-being and its impact on exercise and diabetes.

MENTAL WELL-BEING AND EXERCISE FOR DIABETES MANAGEMENT

The relationship between mental well-being and diabetes management is a critical yet often overlooked aspect. In this chapter, we will explore the connection between exercise, mental health, and diabetes, highlighting the positive impact of physical activity on mental well-being and providing strategies to enhance your mental resilience while managing diabetes. By incorporating strategies to reduce stress, improve motivation, and enhance overall mental well-being, you can optimize your diabetes management and enjoy a more fulfilling and balanced life.

1. The Impact of Exercise on Mental Health:

Exercise has been shown to have numerous mental health benefits for individuals with diabetes. Consider the following ways in which exercise positively impacts mental well-being:

> Stress reduction: Physical activity helps reduce stress levels by promoting the release of endorphins, the

"feel-good" hormones, and providing an outlet for emotional tension.

➢ Mood enhancement: Exercise has a positive impact on mood, promoting feelings of happiness, relaxation, and well-being. It can help alleviate symptoms of anxiety and depression, common among individuals with diabetes.

➢ Improved self-esteem: Engaging in regular exercise can boost self-esteem and confidence, as it provides a sense of accomplishment and body positivity.

➢ Cognitive function and mental clarity: Exercise supports cognitive function and mental clarity, enhancing focus, concentration, and overall cognitive performance.

2. Strategies for Reducing Stress:

Stress management is crucial for overall well-being and diabetes management. Consider the following strategies to reduce stress through exercise:

➢ Mind-body exercises: Engage in mind-body exercises such as yoga, tai chi, or meditation, which promote relaxation, stress reduction, and mindfulness.

➢ Outdoor activities: Spend time in nature and engage in outdoor activities such as hiking, gardening, or cycling, which have a calming and rejuvenating effect on the mind.

➢ Social support: Join exercise groups, classes, or sports teams to benefit from the social support and camaraderie that can help alleviate stress.

3. Enhancing Motivation for Exercise:

Maintaining motivation for exercise can be challenging at times. Consider the following strategies to enhance your motivation:

➢ Set realistic and achievable goals: Set specific, measurable, attainable, relevant, and time-bound (SMART) goals that are meaningful to you. Break them down into smaller milestones and celebrate your achievements along the way.

> Find your "why": Identify the reasons why exercise is important to you and how it aligns with your overall health and well-being goals. Remind yourself of these reasons to stay motivated during challenging times.

> Variety and enjoyment: Engage in a variety of physical activities to keep your workouts interesting and enjoyable. Experiment with different exercises, classes, or outdoor activities to find what you truly enjoy.

4. Building Resilience:

Resilience is essential when managing diabetes and facing its daily challenges. Consider the following strategies to enhance mental resilience:

> Practice self-care: Prioritize self-care activities such as relaxation techniques, mindfulness exercises,

hobbies, or engaging in activities that bring you joy and fulfillment.

➢ Seek support: Reach out to your support system, whether it's friends, family, or support groups. Sharing your experiences and concerns can provide emotional support and valuable insights.

➢ Mindful self-compassion: Cultivate a compassionate and understanding mindset towards yourself. Embrace self-compassion and forgive yourself for any setbacks or perceived failures.

➢ Seek professional help: If you are struggling with significant mental health challenges, don't hesitate to seek professional help from a therapist or counselor who specializes in diabetes and mental well-being.

By recognizing the importance of mental well-being and incorporating strategies to reduce stress, enhance motivation, and build resilience, you can support your diabetes management journey and improve your overall quality of life. In the final chapter, we will provide long-term adherence strategies to help you maintain an active and healthy lifestyle with diabetes.

CONCLUSION

In conclusion, exercise is a powerful tool for managing diabetes and improving overall health and well-being. By incorporating regular physical activity into your routine, you can regulate your blood sugar levels, enhance insulin sensitivity, control weight, and reduce the risk of diabetes-related complications. Throughout this book, we have explored the intricate relationship between exercise and diabetes management, providing practical guidance, and strategies to help you navigate the journey.

We began by understanding the importance of exercise in diabetes management, debunking common myths, and exploring the specific benefits it offers. We then delved into the different types of exercise and provided recommendations for each, including aerobic exercises, strength training, flexibility exercises, and balance training. By understanding how each type of exercise impacts diabetes management, you can tailor your workouts to suit your specific needs and goals.

We addressed the unique considerations for exercise and diabetes, including the role of blood sugar monitoring, adjusting medications, and managing hypoglycemia. By working closely with your healthcare provider and developing an individualized plan, you can exercise safely and effectively while managing your blood sugar levels.

Throughout the book, we also tackled common exercise barriers and provided strategies to overcome them. From lack of motivation and time constraints to fear of hypoglycemia and exercise-related injuries, we explored practical solutions to help you stay on track with your exercise goals. Additionally, we emphasized the importance of nutrition, both pre- and post-exercise, in supporting your workouts and maintaining stable blood sugar levels.

Furthermore, we recognized the profound impact of exercise on mental well-being and provided strategies for reducing stress, enhancing motivation, and building resilience. By nurturing your mental health, you can better navigate the challenges of diabetes management and maintain a positive mindset on your journey.

Lastly, we explored long-term adherence strategies to help you sustain an active and healthy lifestyle with diabetes. By setting realistic goals, finding enjoyment in physical activities, seeking social support, and practicing self-care, you can cultivate habits that promote consistency and long-term success.

As you embark on your exercise and diabetes management journey, remember that it is a continuous process. Be patient with yourself, listen to your body, and make adjustments as needed. Remember to consult with your healthcare provider or a diabetes educator for personalized guidance based on your specific medical condition and individual needs.

By incorporating exercise into your daily life and adopting a holistic approach to diabetes management, you can experience improved blood sugar control, enhanced physical fitness, better mental well-being, and an overall higher quality of life. Stay committed, stay motivated, and embrace the power of exercise as a catalyst for managing your diabetes and achieving optimal health.

www.ingramcontent.com/pod-product-compliance
Lightning Source LLC
Chambersburg PA
CBHW051844250726
48659CB00006B/2021